Menda Brain

By
Neuvare

Copyright

Disclaimer

This book is an activity book, intended for entertainment purposes only.

It is not intended to be used, nor should it be used, to diagnose or treat any medical condition. For diagnosis or treatment of any medical problem, consult your own physician. The editor, publisher and author are not responsible for any specific health or allergy needs that may require medical supervision and are not liable for any damages or negative consequences from any treatment, action, application or preparation, to any person reading or following the information in this book.

Neither is this book intended as a substitute for the medical advice of physicians or therapists. The reader should regularly consult a physician or therapist in matters relating to his/her/their health and particularly with respect to any symptoms that may require diagnosis or medical attention.

This book is designed, based on the author's personal experience and is meant to provide information and motivation to its readers. It is sold with the understanding that the publisher and author are not engaged to render any type of medical, psychological, legal, or any other kind of professional advice.

The content is the sole expression and opinion of its author and publisher. Neither the publisher nor the author shall be liable for any physical, psychological, emotional, financial, or commercial damages, including, but not limited to, special, incidental, consequential or other damages. Our views and rights are the same:

You are responsible for your own choices, actions, and results.

The author and publisher do not assume and hereby disclaim any liability to any party for any loss, damage or disruption caused by information, errors or omissions, whether such information, errors or omissions result from negligence, accident or any other cause

Preface

An active mind is a healthy mind.

Cognitively our brain may need re-training following an injury, sickness or even as we get older. As we age, our brains age with us.

An active brain is a healthy brain and will see us through life and into our golden years.

Surviving a **stroke or Traumatic Brain Injury** is sudden and can occur with no warning. It's like hitting the reset button in your brain.

Sometimes, you are lucky and it's only a soft reboot and things return to normal after some therapy and activity training, whereas on other occasions it may be a hard reboot.

Following a hard reboot, it feels as though your brain is reset to factory default and you have to relearn nearly everything again.

Alzheimer's, dementia, and old age, on the other hand, are progressive diseases and occur over a period of time, short or long. An active brain may not deter these diseases, but it can help to delay the onset.

Unfortunately, with stroke or brain injury. The onset is instant, and the recovery is very long and tedious.

Menda brain books are able to assist, giving you the jump start you need, no matter your level of recovery.

There are different activity levels for every stage of the recovery process, from easy to insane.

The insane level is the ultimate level we would all like to achieve.

We find that this level is very popular among those with youngish brains. wishing to keep their minds as active as possible.

Introduction

An active mind is a healthy mind.

Menda brain books are like having your own personal trainer to keep your brain active.

- Our books are available in two different sizes, with a variety of difficulty levels.

- Our 8.5 x 11 inch is ideal for the elderly or those with brain injuries.
    - Easier to read.
    - Allows you to start at a level you are comfortable with.
    - Begin with the basics and work your way up.

- The 5x8 inch travel version. The ideal size to take with you while travelling.
    - It will easily fit into your purse, backpack, briefcase or coat pocket.
    - Stay active during your subway commutes to and from work.
    - Challenge yourself over lunch or while having coffee.
    - Take it with you on vacation.
    - The options are endless.

*****

Rome was not built in a day, and neither can your brain.

An active brain is a puzzle away.

Table Of Contents

Memory....1

Maths...14

Trace...17

Dot to Dot...27

Coloring In...36

Four in a Row...53

Hitori...65

Word Search...72

Word Puzzle...77

Word Scramble...89

Skyscraper ...91

Maze...98

Solutions...109

How to use this book

Use a pencil when writing in the book.

Start from the begging and progressively work your way through the book.

If you need help, ask someone to assist you.

Depending on the side of the brain that was injured and your cognitive ability, some injuries will require you to re-learn more than others.

You need to learn how to write using your non-dominant hand. Others may require help relearning how to write using their dominant hand.

In either case, we take you step by step through the relearning process.

The same is true for mathematics. We have upped them a notch to make you think. The equations are not difficult and some will require a pen and paper. Try not to use a calculator as this defeats the purpose. It's basic mathematics.

Each puzzle has a purpose. Try your best. No one expects you to be a master at any, but the challenge will help in your recovery.

Follow the process.

Brain fog is a reality and with consistent work, it should begin to subside. By now you should notice a slight difference.

Something to remember though out the recovery process.

The slightest change, no matter how small, is progress.

As you work your way through the book, remember that there are no shortcuts or silly questions.

MEMORY

Study the following pictures one at a time for 30 seconds.
Turn the book over or close it.
Using a separate piece of paper, redraw the picture in as much detail as possible.
Check your percentage in detail in the solution section

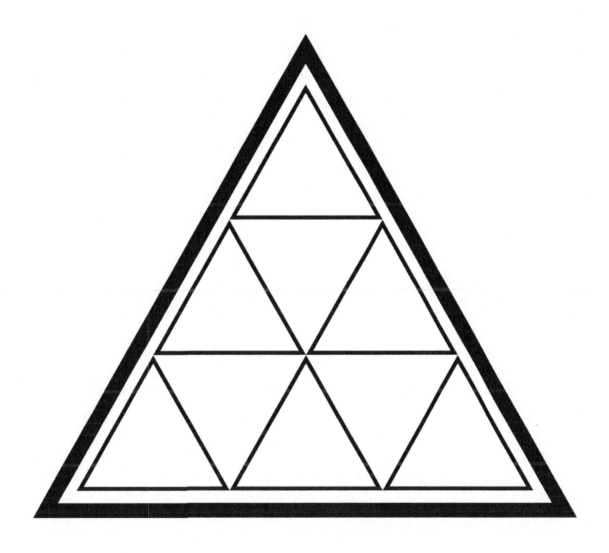

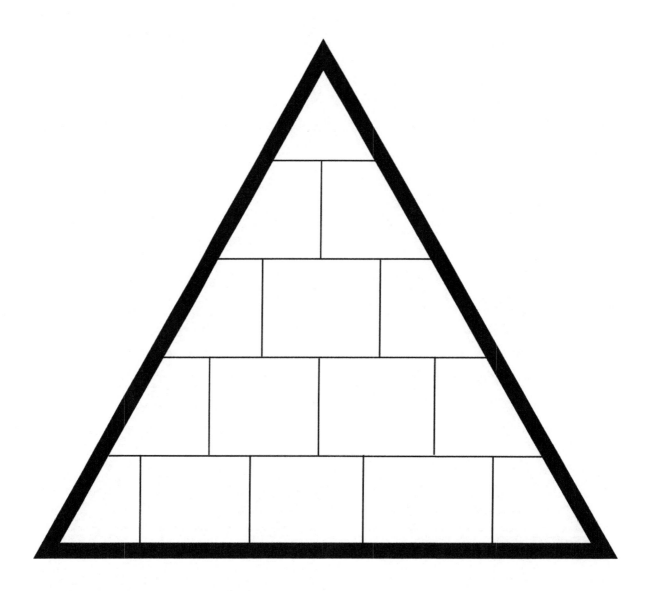

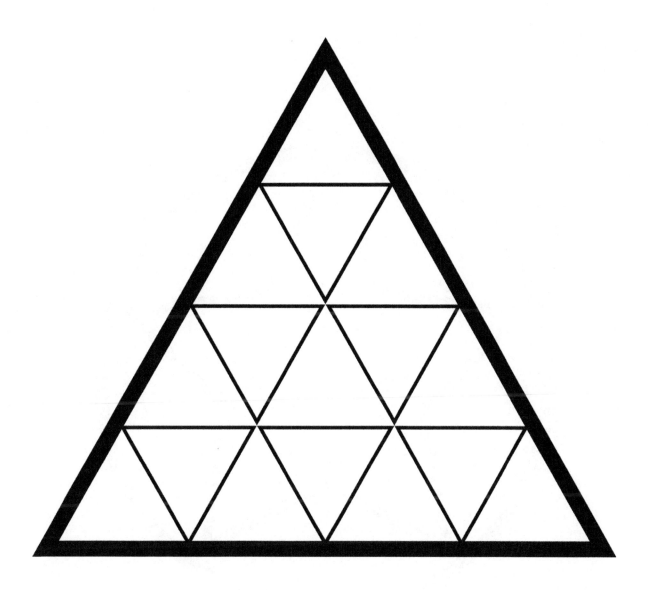

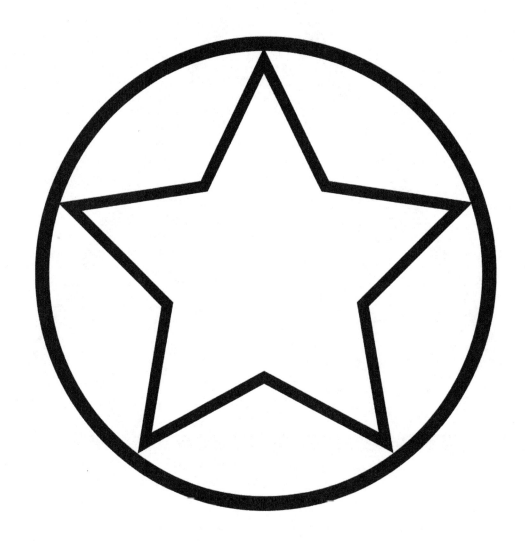

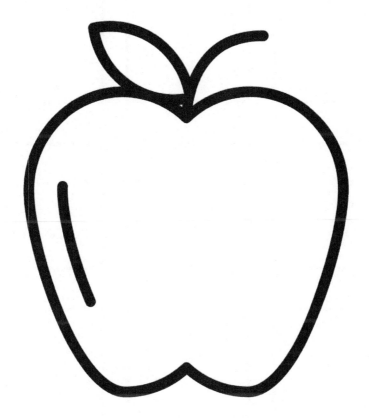

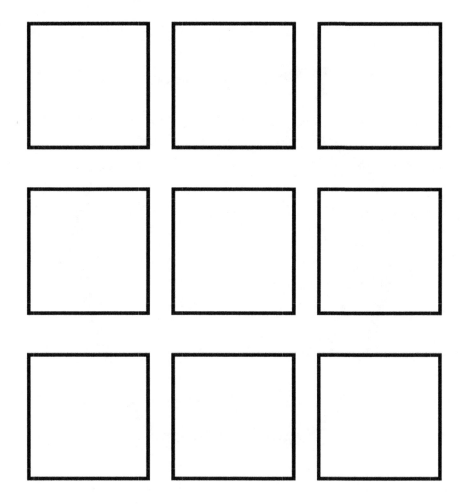

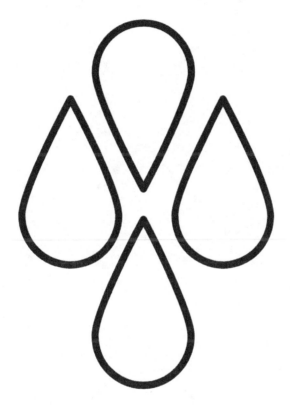

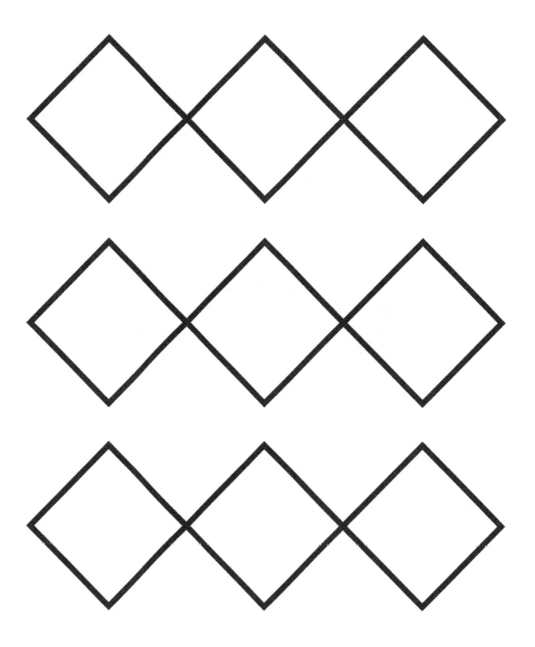

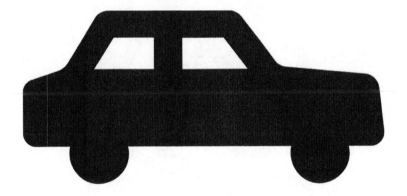

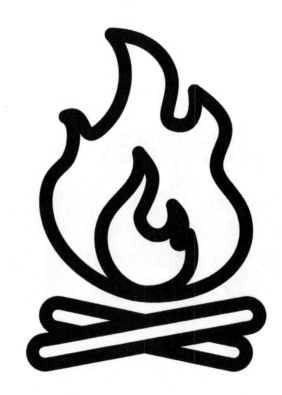

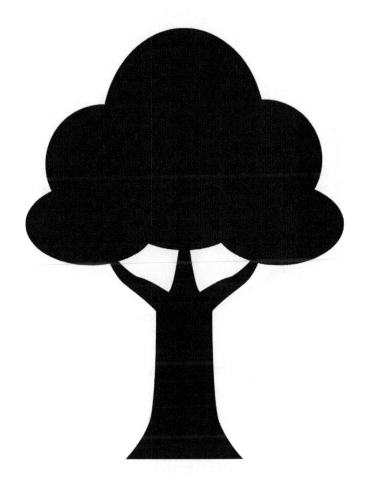

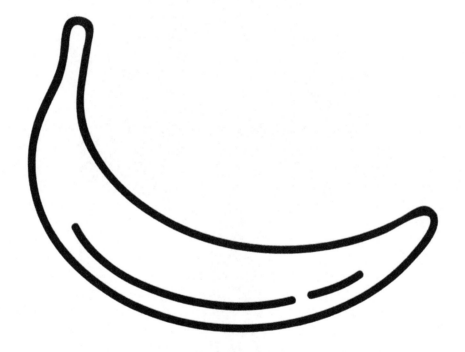